ALPHALIVES WORKSHOP TRAIN®
TEXTS AND MANUALS

CARDIOPULMONARY PROTECTION & RESUSCITATION (CPP&R)

BY

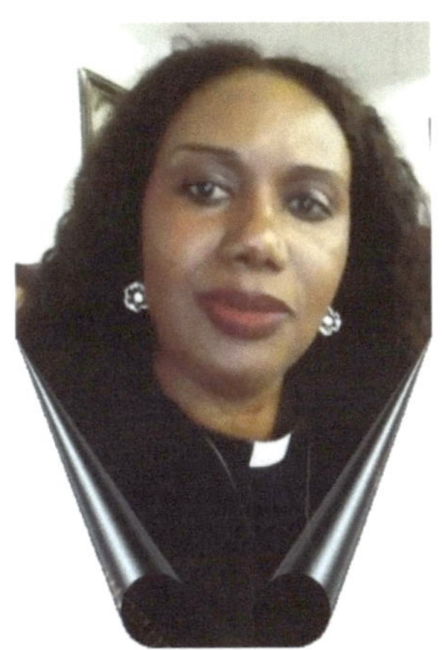

DR. PASTOR
PHIL NGOZI EHIRIM RN. JP.

Prepared as Part of the ACHS Inc. Live-Savers Training Scheme.
Distribution proceeds from this book is channeled to direct healthcare training and
support for vulnerable indigent groups in remote rural communities of Africa.

CARDIOPULMONARY PROTECTION AND RESUSCITATION
- Alphalives Workshop Train Texts and Manuals

1st Edition published (Nigeria, 2005) ALPHALIVES WORKSHOP TRAIN®
2nd Edition published (Nigeria, 2020) ALPHALIVES WORKSHOP TRAIN®

Alphalives Workshop Train is a registered business name of Alpha Charity Healthcare Services Inc.

ISBN 979-858-838-604-3

Author: Dr. Pastor Phil Ngozi Ehirim
Illustrator/Designer: Chuma Mmeka
Pictures: AlphaLives Workshop Train®

©2005 by Alpha Charity Health-Care Services (ACHS) Incorporated

All Rights Reserved.

No part of this handbook may be reproduced or transmitted in any form or by any means, electronic or mechanical, including photocopying, recording or by any information storage and retrieval system, without written permission from the author or her agent.

The information provided within this book is for general learning purposes only. While trying to keep the information up-to-date and correct, there are no representations or warranties, express or implied, about the completeness, accuracy, reliability, suitability or availability with respect to the information contained in this book for any purpose. Any use of this information in life-threatening situations without recourse to a professional, is entirely at your own risk.

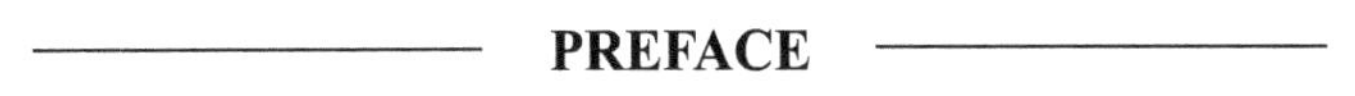

PREFACE

In the less developed world of today, cholera and diarrhea are no longer the major causes of sudden death. Cardiac arrest and stroke, choking, suffocation, trauma, drug overdose, alcoholic intoxication, electrocution, head/neck injuries (such as may occur in an auto or diving accident), etc., are now among the main causes of death. In Africa, there are also a number of other situations induced by civilization, which attack the mind, heart and lungs; bringing about an upsurge in the several reported cases of sudden death.

For nations such as Nigeria, nothing should be more important to the people's welfare of than the continuous development of its health system. The overall socio-economic growth of the country depends first on a strong and healthy workforce.

In a 2004 study conducted by Bishop Iziendu Umeaka Memorial Heart Foundation (a national non-governmental organization) among senior doctors of medicine from 300 public hospitals in Nigeria, it was admitted that every year, more than 400,000 Nigerians (infants, children and adults) are certified 'stone' dead from ailments such as cardiovascular diseases, heart failure, and choking. Of that number, about 80% are believed to have died as a result of the lack of practical CPR knowledge within the family, community and among healthcare workers and medical personnel. The situation is heightened by the lack of an Emergency Medical Services (EMS) System in local Nigerian communities.

The resultant stress brought about by the prevalent hardship and citizens' struggle to survive in the Nigeria of today, will mean according to the professionals, the certified death of more than 4.5 million persons from cardiopulmonary failure within the next 10 years.

This number can be effectively reduced by about 50% if the nation embarks on a massive public enlightenment programme on cardiovascular diseases and related conditions, and training of its citizenry in CPR. It is also pertinent that the government establishes an EMS System in local communities.

The all-essential nature of CPR, the need for the people to practice it and cultivate healthier lifestyles to protect their hearts and lungs must be effectively communicated to the Nigerian people.

No meaningful development in the Nigerian public health system, can be achieved without the effective teaching of professionals like nurses in the subject known as CPR; using less technical terms and illustrations. For the first time in sub-Saharan Africa, this essential and activity has finally been initiated by **ACHS Inc.**

We have taken some great pains in this work because we know that effective teaching of the subject, cannot be made from the confines of clinical or laboratory conditions only. The primer written by a medical academician may have its place in teaching the subject to students with extensive medical knowledge, but we are aware that it is out of place in the unbridled teaching of student nurses and other healthcare workers.

What is needed is a handy and practical book jam packed with relevant information, techniques and procedures, which are field tested, workable and unencumbered by tongue twisting medical terminology or jargon. This book is designed to fulfill these stringent demands.

Best of all, it is an authoritative book written by an outstanding international Intensive Care Unit Nurse, Cardiopulmonary Resuscitation Expert (Member, American Hearts Association) and Primary Healthcare Researcher with bias for Preventive Medicine in Africa. When Phil Ngozi Ehirim talks about the subject matter of this text, she is no theorist pontificating from the aesthetic confines of an ivory tower.

Phil is one of the twelve master public training instructors in the world. For over twenty-five years, she has been a leading producer and famous columnist/public trainer on health issues for a number of newspapers columns and radio/television programs. Her charity health organization ACHS Inc. is a legendary example of both creative resource/capacity building and effective public health management. The organization is also an international dutiful employer of healthcare professionals including specialist doctors, registered nurses, and public/community health education experts.

ALPHA CHARITY HEALTHCARE SERVICES (ACHS) INC is an international membership-based, non-governmental charity organization. Founded in Texas U.S.A. 2001 as a non-profit; and further incorporated in Nigeria as an N.G.O. in 2003. Its main focus is the provision of Free Healthcare, Medical Services, Education and Counseling to underprivileged persons. We uplift the quality of life and overall well-being of disadvantaged Nigerians, especially youths, women and children; the indigent, the physically challenged, the old, and people living with HIV/AIDS.

We have continued to achieve our organizational goals through the establishment of FREE Rural Health Clinic in various Local Government Areas of Nigeria. We have also since inception, facilitated a FREE Helpless Patients Home Visit Scheme, and instituted Voluntary HIV Counseling and Testing (VCT) Centers. Most importantly, is our Public Education Programme (PEP) through the mass media and workshops programmes that cut across borders. Today, Alpha Charity is the foremost organization in Africa to develop and establish a national Health Development Project to train potential responders to revive victims of choking and sudden death; and to prevent the occurrence of diseases tagged: ALPHALIVES WORKSHOP TRAIN®

Besides this workshop texts and manuals series, Phil has written several articles which appear in leading medical journals, public health education and preventive medicine publications.

Please support us in any way you can, to help us reach many more of the unreached and vulnerable persons in the heart of Africa. You may call: +234 803 335 7413 to find out how; or visit www.acamph.org for more details.

Chuma Mmeka *(Illustrator, Designer)*
Chief Operating Officer (C.O.O), Alpha Charity Healthcare Services Inc.

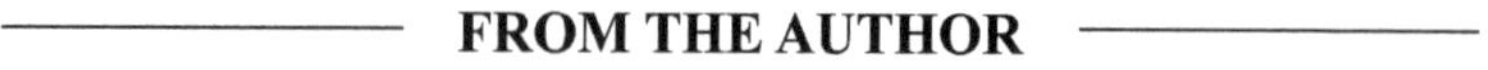

FROM THE AUTHOR

This work is my response to a popular demand from the thousands of participants in Nigeria, Africa (especially the First Aid & Healthcare Providers) who while benefitting from my public teaching exercises, also need a handy material from the lessons to help answer their questions whenever the need arises.

This edition has been carefully laid out in several parts to accommodate most recent and relevant information on sundry issues connected to cardiovascular health and how to revive victims of choking or sudden death. Other relevant issues like the implications of stress and depression, headaches, hypertension; their interrelationships and deadly effects; plus, actions for survival are also treated in this work.

I hereby acknowledge the American Hearts Association whose relentless activities in the United States first and foremost, provided the inspiration and first technical information used in the development of this work.

I am particularly grateful to all those too numerous to mention, including my darling husband Vincent who is equally a nurse, my lovely children, extended family and congregation who pray with me; professional colleagues who have contributed to my knowledge base in one way or the other; and my fans and beneficiaries from across the globeithout whom we could have gained no traction in this vision. I want to thank in a special way, Chuma Mmeka my erstwhile manager and now C.O.O of ACHS Inc. in Africa for helping me with the preparation of this manuscript.

Thank you all. Your constructive criticisms, knowledge and personal involvements all made this book a success. May God bless you all. I cannot thank you enough, but I can say:

"KEEP SMILING, DON'T WORRY, BE HAPPY"

Pastor Dr. Phil Ngozi Ehirim RN. JP. *(Author)*
Founder / President, Alpha Charity Healthcare Services Inc.

INTRODUCING CPP&R

CARDIOPULMONARY PROTECTION & RESUSCITATION (CPP&R) is a novel and exclusive manual developed to describe in practical details, the need to protect the human heart and its vessels; whose heart and breathing can be affected; how to prevent diseases from wrecking the system, and the simple steps in reviving victims of sudden death. It is prepared in line with the training curriculum of the **ALPHALIVES WORKSHOP TRAIN.®**

The ALPHALIVES WORKSHOP TRAIN has continued to generate tremendous local and international media publicity. The Workshop Train Text, which is the **first of its kind in Nigeria particularly and Africa as a whole,** provides the student nurse, healthcare provider, caregiver, families and individuals with the most relevant and recent information to maintain a healthy heart. It also deals with whose heart could be impaired and when; while at the same time, equipping the user with the practical skills training required to revive victims of sudden death also known as Cardiopulmonary Resuscitation (CPR), and victims of choking also known as Heimlich Maneuver.

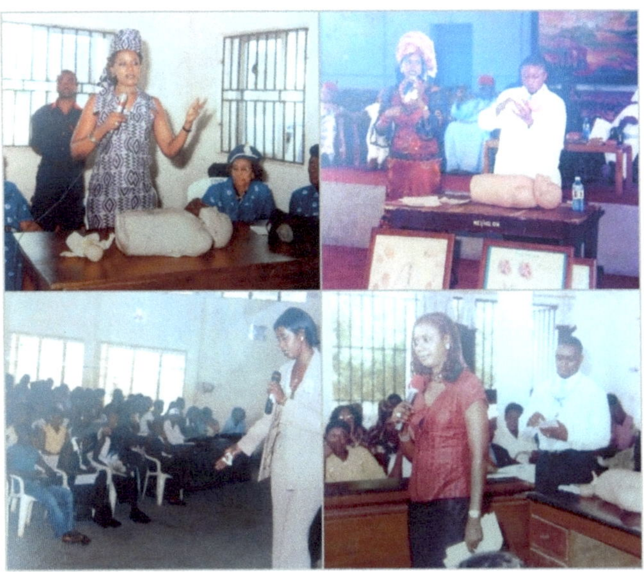

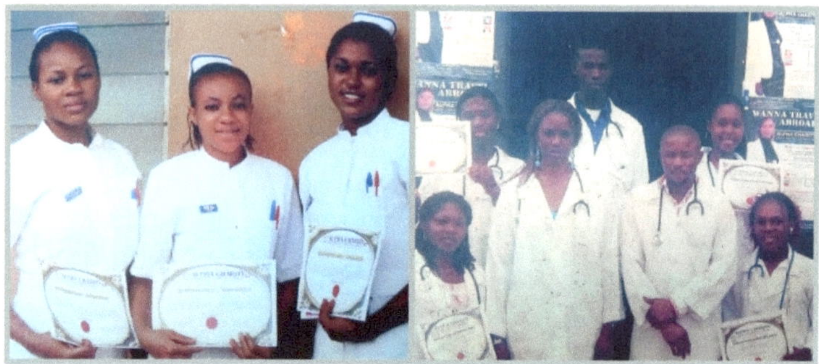

This unique meeting point, benefiting both the healthcare worker/student and the "layperson" is the only panacea to the number of certified deaths from cardiovascular diseases and heart/breath failure within individual families in the African community. The workshop train is moving throughout Africa, beginning with the Nigerian Federation to effectively establish the all-important public health development initiative.

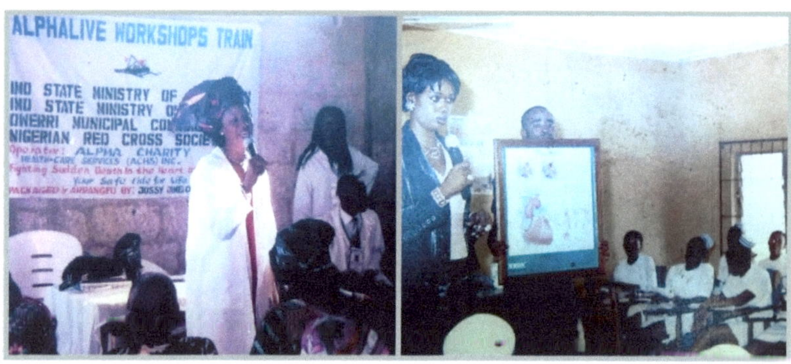

The book Cardiopulmonary Protection & Resuscitation (CPP&R) tells the ordinary person who reads it the "how to" and "when to" protect or resuscitate a person's heart - from spelling out the objectives to inspiring the reader in action.

It is a practical book filled with useful information. It is quite a timely book containing the latest techniques and simple steps of protecting the

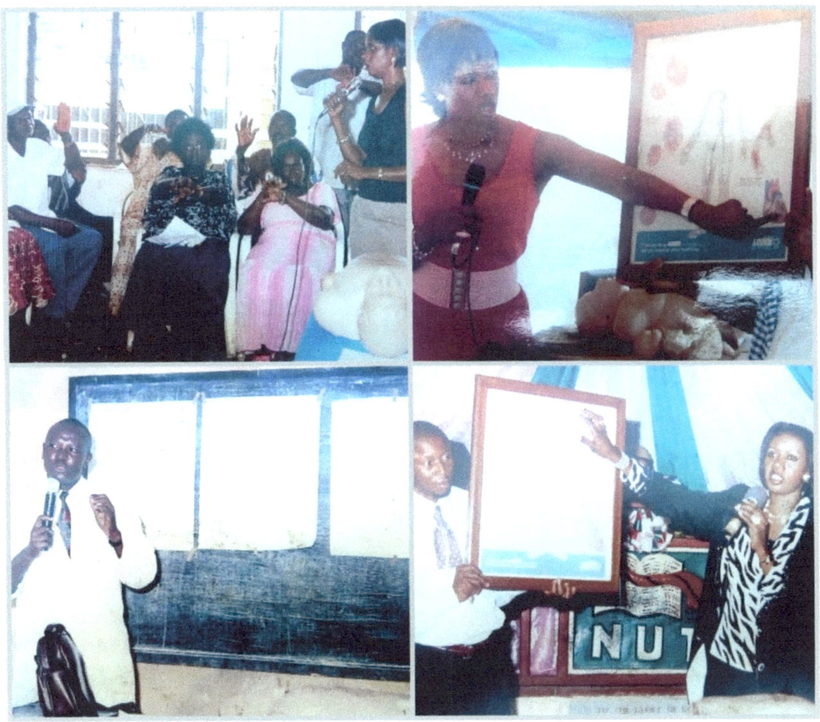

human body from heart related diseases and how to resuscitate a victim of choking or sudden death as a result of heart attack, stroke, coma, electrocution, choking, trauma, epilepsy, suffocation, smoke/gas inhalation, drug over dose, alcoholic intoxication, head/neck injury (such as may occur in an automobile or diving accident), etc. Among all the likely causes of sudden death, cardiac arrest, choking and stoke are the most common.

THE NORMAL HEART AND LUNG

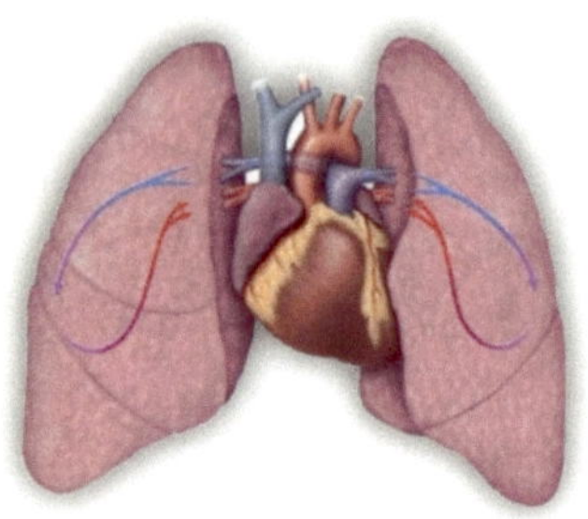

The heart is a muscle about the size of a clenched fist. It is located in the center of the chest behind the breastbone (sternum) and in front of the spine. The coronary arteries supply blood to the heart. The right side of the heart receives blood from the body through the coronary arteries and pumps it through the pulmonary artery to the lungs where it picks up oxygen. The left side of the heart receives oxygen-rich blood from the lungs and pumps it through the aorta to the body.

The function of the heart is to pump blood to the lungs, where it picks up oxygen, and then to the rest of the body, where it delivers the oxygen. The adult heart pumps approximately 5 liters of blood per minute. All the cells of the body require oxygen to carry out their natural assignments. When the heart stops pumping the blood, cardiac arrest is said to have occurred and oxygen is no longer circulated. As a result, the oxygen stored in the brain and other vital organs is used up quickly. The heartbeat is triggered by natural electrical impulses sent through the heart 60 to 100 times per minute in a healthy, resting adult. During exercises, the heart of the average person can pump up to 25 liters each minute.

The lungs consist of several tiny air sacs called alveoli and surrounded by small blood vessels called capillaries. Nerve impulses from the brain to the chest muscles and the diaphragm cause a person to breathe. With each breath, air is carried through the airway (i.e. nose, mouth, throat, larynx, trachea, and bronchi) and on into the air sacs of the lungs. When the airsacs are filled with the oxygenated air, oxygen then enters the blood in the vessels surrounding the air sacs. The oxygenated blood returns to the heart, which then pumps it throughout the body.

As oxygen is taken is taken from the blood by the cells in the body, carbon dioxide is given off as a waste product. Carbon dioxide is carried by the blood back to the air sacs and is exhaled out of the body. When air is inhaled, the blood uses up ¼ of the oxygen, the rest is exhaled.

This is why mouth-to-mouth breathing can provide the victim with adequate oxygen. When breathing stops respiratory arrest is said to have occurred. The heart continues to pump blood for several minutes, carrying existing stores of oxygen to the brain and other parts of the body. Early, prompt rescue efforts for the victim of respiratory arrest or choking can often prevent the victim's heart from stopping.

HEART PROTECTION:

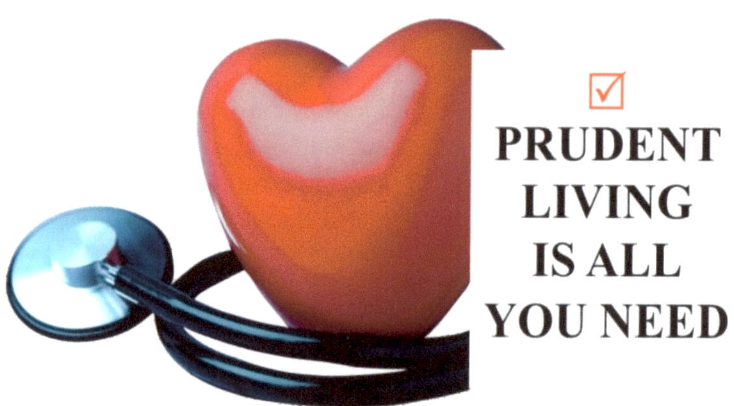

Prudent heart living is a lifestyle that may minimize the risk of future heart disease. A good number of adult Africans are overweight, lead sedentary lives, and smoke heavily. Many have high levels of cholesterol and other fatty substances in their blood, and high blood pressure is common. Millions of Nigerians develop unhealthy living habits during childhood that endangers their hearts for life.

Some children begin early in life to over-eat and to develop a taste for foods high in cholesterol and calories. Some children do not get enough exercise (for example, they may be busy watching too much television). Smoking frequently begins in the early teens, and children are more likely to smoke if their parents or adults around them do.

Reducing risk factors may reduce the risk of having a heart attack or stroke. At the very least, reducing the risks can result in good general health and physical fitness and can benefit every member of the family. Children stand to benefit most by learning the habits of prudent heart living early in life.

The following pages describe in simple detail five specific ways that prudent heart living can be established and maintained.

1.   Cigarette Smoking? SAY NO!

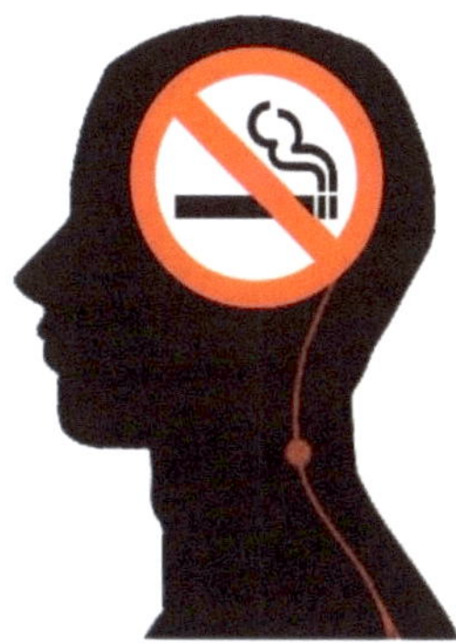

Exposure to cigarette smoke is the most important single cause of preventable deaths in Nigeria. Cigarette smokers have a greater risk of dying from a variety of diseases than do non-smokers; and they have more than twice the risk of heart attacks and two to four times the risk of sudden cardiac death.

If you have been a heavy smoker, will it help to stop now? Yes. People who quit smoking have a rapidly reduced risk of heart disease, and after a period of years their death rate is nearly as low as that of people who never smoked.

The earlier a person begins to smoke or use tobacco in any form, the greater the risk to future health. There is considerable peer pressure on teenagers to use tobacco, and whether they resist may depend largely on the example set by their parents and adults around them.

Inhalation of environmental tobacco smoke, that is, passive smoking, has also been associated with an increased risk of smoking-related diseases.

In developed nations like the United States, public buildings, hospitals, and many restaurants and businesses have implemented firm nonsmoking policies. These efforts encourage their patrons and employees to recognize risks for both active and passive smokers.

Ongoing efforts by the ALPHLIVES WORKSHOP TRAIN in the area of public health should encourage a decrease in the number of deaths and disability from cigarette smoking in Nigeria.

TOBACCO DESTROYS: A Sure killer

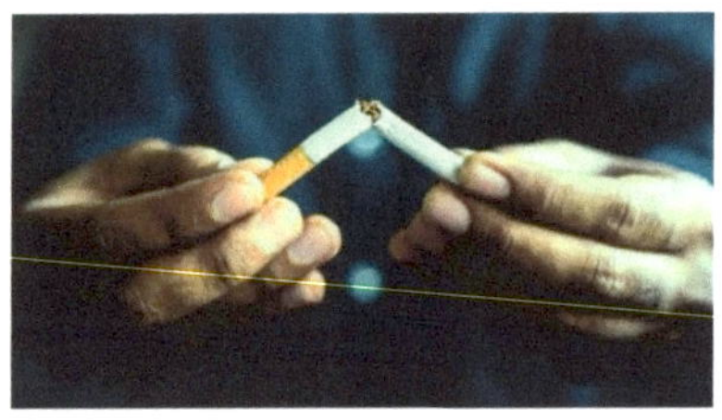

For years the link between cigarette and cigar smoking and lung cancer and lung disease has been well known. Most people still associate smoking with breathing problems. But that's not the whole story. Smoking is also a major cause of heart disease and stroke. The fact is, every year more than 100,000 deaths in Nigeria are due to smoking. Another 100,000 of deaths are due to heart and blood vessel diseases.

Environmental Tobacco Smoke: Smokers aren't the only ones affected by tobacco smoke. Environmental Tobacco Smoke (ETS) also called passive smoke or second hand smoke, is a serious health hazard for non-smokers, especially children. ETS contains more than 4,000 chemical and at least 40 known cancer-causing chemical agents.

Non-smokers who have high blood pressure or high blood cholesterol have an even greater risk of developing heart disease when they are exposed to secondhand smoke. Environmental Tobacco Smoke causes about 10 times as many cardiovascular deaths as cancer deaths. Studies show that the risk of death from heart disease is about 30 percent higher among people exposed to environmental tobacco smoke at home or work.

Secondhand smoke promotes illness too. In 1996 according to available research, about 11 million children up to age 18 (more that 20 percent of

all Nigerian children) were exposed to ETS in the home. Children of smokers have many more respiratory infections than do children of nonsmokers. Non-smoking women exposed to tobacco smoke are also more likely to have low-birth-weight babies. The best way to safeguard your health is to avoid tobacco smoke as much as you can.

Smoking and Circulation: Smoking or being exposed to high amounts of environmental tobacco smoke causes several temporary effects on a person's heart and blood vessels. The nicotine in the smoke temporarily increases the blood pressure, the heart rate, the amount of blood pumped by the heart and the blood flow in the heart's arteries. It also causes the arteries in the arms and legs to constrict.

Smoking doesn't cause high blood pressure, but it does increase the risk of developing cardiovascular disease in people with high blood pressure. Nicotine isn't the only bad element in cigarette smoke. Carbon monoxide gets in the blood and reduces the oxygen available to the heart and all other parts of the body. Tobacco smoke makes blood clot faster and makes clots more likely to form. These effects harm a person's cardiovascular system.

Smoking and Stroke: Several large studies have linked cigarette smoking with different kinds of stroke. In the Framingham Heart Study, stroke incidence was 40 percent higher in male smokers and 60 percent higher in women smokers than in non-smokers. Within two years of quitting smoking, stroke risk fell significantly. Within five years stroke risk was the same as for non-smokers.

Smoking and Chronic Lung Disease: Smoking is the main cause of chronic bronchitis and emphysema. These chronic lung diseases put more pressure on the heart and when heart disease is present, may result in heart failure. Secondhand smoke is also a problem, especially for children. Each year it causes up to 300,000 chest and throat infections (such as pneumonia and bronchitis) in children less than one and a half years old. Up to 15,000 of them end up hospitalized.

Smoking and Teenagers: The earlier a person starts smoking, the greater the risk to their health in the future. Among teenagers, the risk of heart attack in later life seems remote. But even teenagers can suffer coughing, lower stamina and a fast heart rate from smoking.

These conditions will worsen over time and can develop into heart disease or chronic lung disease if a person keeps smoking. Most smokers start smoking as teenagers. In fact, it's estimated that 80 percent of all smokers start smoking before age 18. 3,000 young people under age 18 start smoking every day and 1,000 of them will eventually die from cardiovascular disease.

Smoking and The Birth Control Pill: Women smokers using oral contraceptives have higher risks of heart attack and stroke than non-smokers who use the pill. Smoking and taking birth control pills also increases the risk of narrowed blood vessels (peripheral vascular disease).

Low-Tar and Low-Nicotine Cigarettes: No cigarettes are safe. Scientists have found no evidence that smoking low-tar and low-nicotine cigarettes make smoking any safer. In fact, smokers of low-tar, low-nicotine cigarettes smoke more cigarettes and inhale more deeply to make up for the reduced nicotine. This can create new problems, because tar and nicotine aren't the only harmful substances in tobacco smoke. By inhaling more deeply, smokers take in more of the other harmful substances and may increase their risk of disease.

Stop Smoking Now!

No matter how much or how long you have smoked, when you quit smoking, your risk of heart disease starts to drop. One year after quitting, your risk of death from heart attack is cut in half. It is important to stop smoking before the signs of heart disease appear. Once they show up, even if you quit smoking, it will take 15 years for your heart attack risk to get as low as someone who's never smoked. Don't wait until you have heart disease or a stroke to quit.

Quit while you are still ahead.

2. High Blood Pressure

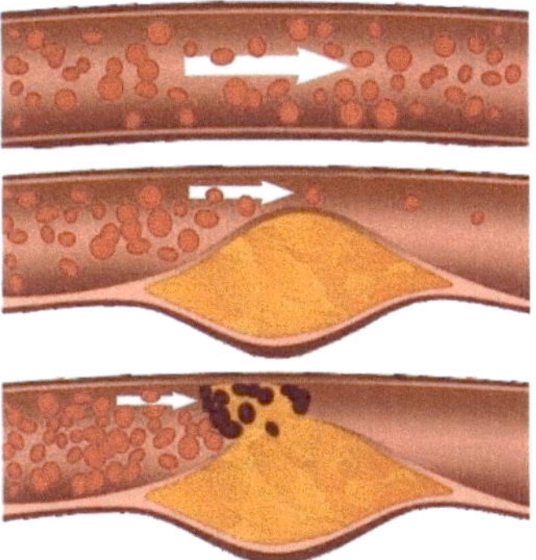

Uncontrolled high blood pressure (hypertension) is associated with a greater risk of heart attack. When hypertension is not treated, it becomes a major health problem and the result may be damage to blood vessels in the heart, kidneys and other organs.

High blood pressure increases the risk of stroke, heart attack, and kidney failure. When high blood pressure is combined with other risk factors, such as obesity, exposure to cigarette smoke, high blood cholesterol levels, physical inactivity, or diabetes, the risk of heart attack or stroke is also greatly increased.

The underlying cause of high blood pressure in most patients is still unknown. However, high blood pressure is usually controllable. Treatment includes diet changes and increased exercise. Drugs to lower the blood pressure may be used if dieting and exercise are irregular. People who know they have high blood pressure can guard against its most harmful effects by going for regular medical checkups.

3.   Saturated Fat & Cholesterol in the Diet is Dangerous for You
Cholesterol is a substance manufactured by our bodies. It is also present in the foods we eat. It is found in all animal products and is especially high in egg yolks and organ meats (liver, kidneys and brains). When excess cholesterol is deposited on the inner walls of arteries, it leads to a narrowing of the blood vessels known as *atherosclerosis.*

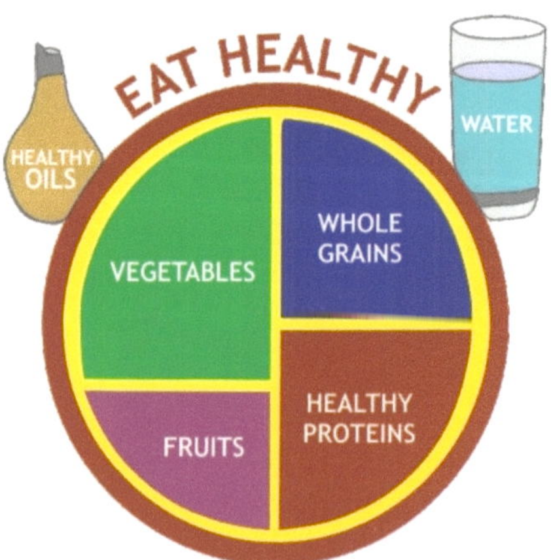

Saturated fats, such as those in red meats, butter, cheese, cream and whole milk, also seem to help raise the blood's cholesterol level. On the other hand, partially substituting polyunsaturated fats (such as liquid vegetable oils, with the exception of coconut and palm kernel oil, which are examples of saturated fats) lowers cholesterol levels in most people.

The goal is to keep the saturated fat content of the diet low. You cannot eliminate saturated fat entirely. It is present in many of the foods you eat. However, you can reduce the amount of saturated fat in your diet if you follow these recommendations:

- Have fish and poultry for most of your meals.
- Cook poultry without the skin.
- When you serve red meat (beef, pork, veal and lamb), use lean cuts, trim off excess fat and serve small portions.
- Cook with limited amounts of liquid vegetable oils and poly-unsaturated margarine.
- Use skim-milk products.
- Eat no more than three egg yolks per week. Use "egg substitutes" where possible.
- Use low-fat cooking methods such as baking, broiling, and roasting: avoid fried foods.

Dietary change should never be drastic. You can harm yourself by cutting out essential foods. A faddish diet can lead to other health problems. However, with moderate changes in your diet, regular exercises and careful attention to your intake of cholesterol and saturated fats, you can usually keep blood cholesterol down to normal levels.

4.   Regular Exercises

Evidence suggests that men who lead sedentary lives may have a higher risk of heart attack than those who get regular, vigorous exercises. Exercise tones the muscles, stimulates circulation, helps prevent excess weight, and promotes a general feeling of well-being. The survival rate of heart attack victims is higher in those who have exercised regularly than in those who have not.

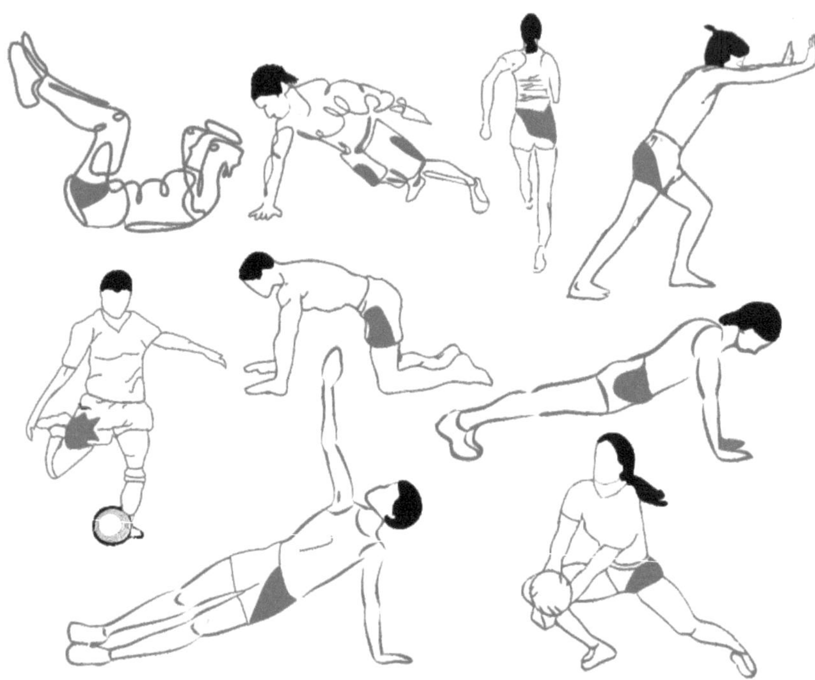

This does not mean that you should go about digging up hard ground or play a hard game at weightlifting if you are not used to such exertion. Before starting an exercise program or heavy physical labor, consult your physician. He or she may suggest an exercise test to evaluate your physical or heart condition.

When participating in an exercise program, you should always increase your physical activity gradually. Walk briskly when it is not absolutely necessary to ride. Take up a sport you will enjoy if your doctor says you are fit for it.

5.   Count Your Calories To Control Your Weight
Most people reach their normal adult weight between the ages of 21 and 25. With each year after that, fewer calories are needed to maintain this

weight. But people in their 30s and 40s often eat as much as they did in their early 20s, and if they become less active, the excess calories are stored as fat.

Life expectancy may be shorter for people who are overweight. Middle-aged men who are much overweight, for example, have about three times the risk of a fatal heart attack more than middle-aged men of normal weight. Obesity also increases the risk of high blood pressure, high cholesterol and diabetes.

There is no quick, easy way to reduce. It is best to avoid extreme reducing diets because they usually leave out foods essential to good health. Even when these diets lower weight, they do not help you develop eating habits that will keep weight normal. Controlling the fat in your diet may allow you to maintain an appropriate body weight. If you need to reduce, ask your doctor or diet specialist for advice.

SIGNALS AND RISK FACTORS

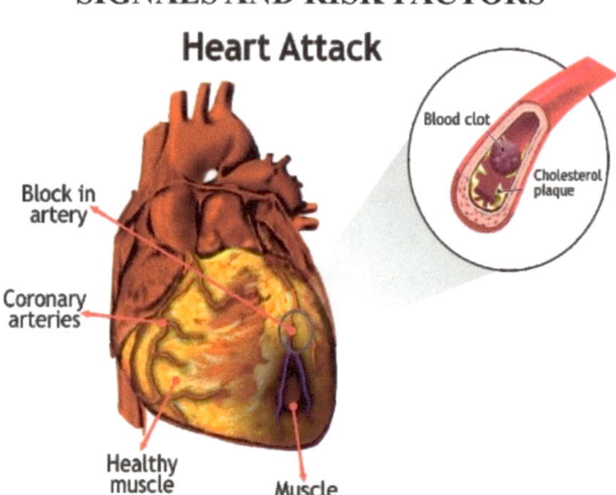

Several factors increase a person's chances of having heart attack. Some risk factors can be changed or controlled, others cannot. The danger of heart attack increases with the number of risk factors - the more risk factors present, the greater the risk. Reducing risk factors, however, can slow down arterial disease and even reverse it.

Men have an increased risk of heart attack more than women; but it is important for women to control changeable risk factors as well. A woman's chance of dying after a heart attack is greater than a man's, and heart disease is the leading cause of death in women.

Major risk factors that cannot be changed
- Heredity
- Male gender
- Increasing age

Major risk factors that can be changed
- Cigarette smoke
- High blood pressure
- Physical inactivity

Other Contributing Factors
- Diabetes
- Obesity
- Stress
- Elevated blood sugar levels (diabetes) can be controlled, but the increased risk of heart disease cannot be eliminated.

How to Recognize a Heart Attack:
When someone suffers a heart attack, minutes - especially the first few minutes- essentially count. Knowing the signals more often than not saves lives.

Chest discomfort is the most common sign of a heart attack with the following characteristics:
- Uncomfortable pressure, fullness, squeezing, or pain in the center of the chest behind the breastbone.
- It may spread to or occasionally originate in the shoulder, the neck, the lower jaw or either arm.

Other signs of a heart attack may include any, all, or none of the following:
- Chest discomfort with lightheadedness
- Fainting
- Sweating
- Nausea
- Shortness of breath

Not all these warning signs occur in every heart attack. If some start to occur however, don't wait. Get help immediately. Delay may be deadly! Because the victim may not act in his or her own best interest, it is essential that the nearest person calls for help immediately and be prepared to perform cardiopulmonary resuscitation (CPR) if necessary. If you are with someone who is having the signals of a heart attack and if they last longer than a few minutes, act at once.

The first step after calling for help, (or in the event of its establishment,

activating the EMS system) should be to have the victim rest quietly and calmly. Because both angina pectoris and heart attack are caused by too little oxygen to the heart muscles, the victim's activity and fear must be kept to a minimum. The victim should be allowed to assume the position that gives him or her most comfort and allows the easiest breathing.

Actions for Survival:
- Recognize the signals.
- Stop whatever you're doing and sit or lie down.
- If the signals last more than a few minutes, get help and take the victim to the nearest hospital with emergency cardiac care equipment.

STROKE: SIGNALS AND RISK FACTORS

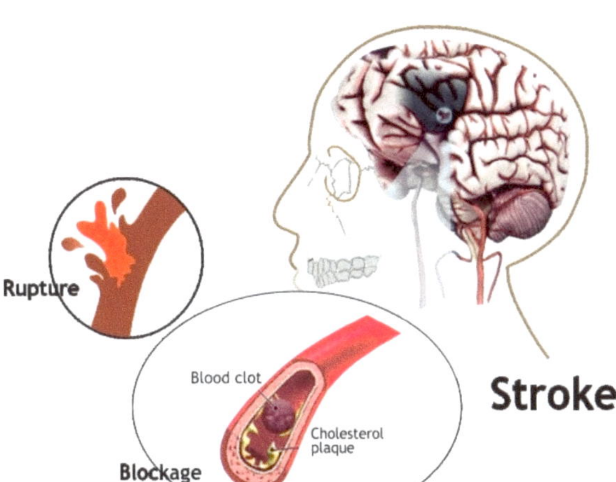

Signals of Stroke:

Stroke is a common and serious brain illness of sudden onset. It results from the blockage or rupture of a blood vessel. Most often strokes are caused by a blood clot in an artery. Stroke is the leading cause of death and disability within sub-Saharan Africa, especially in Nigeria.

Strokes may precipitate conditions that require rescue breathing, chest compression, or both. Though most common in older people, strokes happen in persons of all ages. You should know the early warning signs of stroke so that emergency care can be started promptly.

Warning signs or symptoms of stroke may include the following:
- Sudden weakness or numbness of the face, arm, or leg on one side of the body
- Loss of speech, slurred or incoherent speech
- Unexplained dizziness, unsteadiness, or sudden falls
- Dimness or loss of vision, particularly in one eye
- Loss of consciousness

An unusually severe or sudden intense headache can be an important warning sign of a brain hemorrhage. These warning signs may be temporary (a transient ischemic attack or TIA), lasting less than 24 hours or sometimes just a few minutes. When one occurs, a physician's attention should be sought immediately since prompt medical or surgical treatment can prevent the stroke.

Although similar signs may result from alcohol or drug intoxication, insulin reactions, or other disease, they may also be signs of stroke, even when temporary. Successful treatment of the victim is linked to early recognition, call for help and rapid transport to the hospital. The fundamentals of basic life support are important in the care of a patient with stroke, particularly when consciousness is impaired. Airway obstruction can occur. If it does, immediately open the airway and perform rescue breathing.

RISK FACTORS FOR STROKE:

Risk factors that cannot be controlled -
•**Age:** The incidence of stroke more than doubles every 10 years for people older than 55 years.
•**Gender:** Men have a greater risk of stroke than women. Women, who take oral contraceptives, especially if they also smoke, have a greater risk than other women.
•**Race:** Members of the black race have a greater risk of stroke than the white race.
•**Diabetes**
•**Prior stroke**
•**Heredity**

Risk factors that can be controlled -
•**High Blood Pressure:** Hypertension is the most important risk factor for stroke because it affects one in every three Africans, yet it is usually readily controlled. The higher the blood pressures, the greater the risk. Much of the decline in the incidence of stroke is the awareness created for

an improved management of high blood pressure.
•**Heart Disease:** A diseased heart can be both a defective (weak) pump and a source of blood clots. Some risk factors for coronary heart disease like elevated cholesterol level are direct risk factors for stroke.
•**Cigarette Smoking**
•**High red blood cell count:** An increase in the red blood cell count is a risk factor for stroke. The reason is that increased red blood cells thicken the blood and make clot formations more likely.
•**Transient Ischemic Attacks:** TIAs are stroke like symptoms that disappear in less than 24 hours. TIAs are extremely important; they are strong predictors of stroke. They are usually treated with drugs that help keep clots from forming.

Practical Cardiopulmonary Resuscitation

CPR is short for Cardiopulmonary Resuscitation. *Cardio* in the word here represents the circulation of blood by the heart in a human being. *Pulmonary* represents breathing while *Resuscitation* simply means to bring back to live.

CPR is administered when someone's breathing or pulse (or both) stops. When both stop, sudden death has occurred. Sudden death could be said to have several causes including poisoning, drowning, choking, suffocation, electrocution and smoke inhalation - but the most common is heart attack.

Everyone should know the signals of heart attack and the actions for survival. They should also have a plan for emergency action.

To make for easier understanding, we shall treat CPR in a practical dimension.

The ABCs of CPR
CPR is a practical skill technique that is always said to be as simple as ABC: A is for Airway, B is for Breathing, while C is for Circulation. To effectively utilize this ABC Technique, the potential resuscitator must work on the victim of sudden death within 6 minutes of the incident. (S)he must act definitely and fast before it becomes too late.

After 6 - 8minutes, the Resuscitator might only just succeed in reviving a living individual no better than a vegetable; or lose the victim after all. It is also important that the resuscitator considers the situation at hand within a split second before acting. For example, if the victim was a helpless invalid bedridden for a long period, suffering from a medical ailment that naturally and finally leads to a long awaited death, then there should be no need to resist its occurrence.

To begin with, the resuscitator must first assess the victim. If the person isn't responsive, the next action will be to get help. (Activate the Local Emergency Medical Services System or call the Local Ambulance/Hospital number; or call for a car with which to take the victim to the nearest hospital). Then begin the ABC Technique of CPR: Airway, Breathing and Circulation.

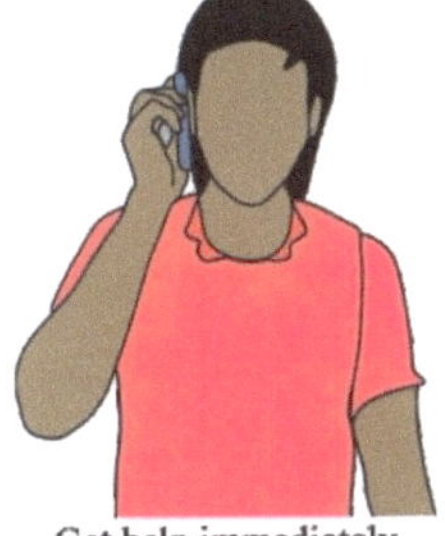

Get help immediately

Assessment and Activation
If you find an adult who has collapsed, you should first, assess the victim. Find out if he or she is unresponsive by gently shaking a shoulder and shouting "Are you all right?" If the person doesn't respond to you, call out for help. If a helper is available, let the person know about the emergency and try to get help. If no one else is available, make the necessary calls yourself. When you return, first loosen all tight fastenings on the victim (if any). Where this could prove difficult, discard the idea and continue with the main task at hand.

Begin the ABCs: Airway, Breathing and Circulation.
A.   <u>A</u>irway
To open the airway, gently lift the victim's chin with one hand while pushing down on the forehead with your other hand. You want to tilt the head back. Once the airway is open, lean over and put your ear close to the victim's mouth.

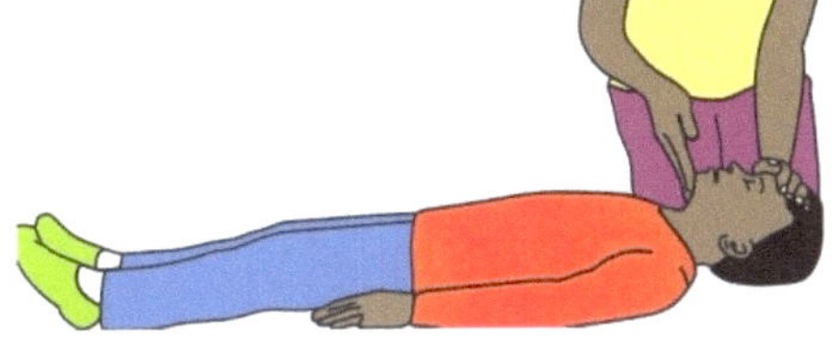

- Look at the chest for movement.
- Listen for the sound of breathing.
- Feel for breath on your cheek.

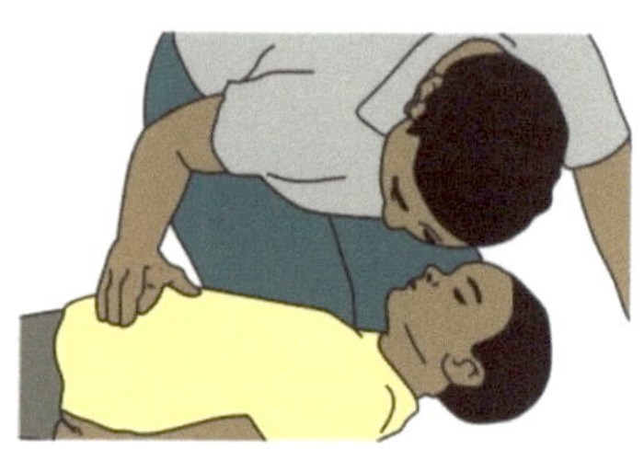

If the victim is breathing, roll the person onto his or her side as a unit (this is called the recovery position).

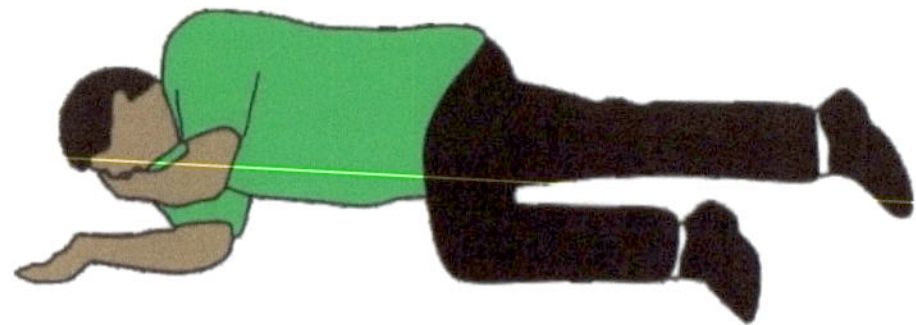

If none of these signs is present, the person is not breathing and will require help to do that. If opening the airway does not cause the person to spontaneously start breathing, you will have to provide rescue breathing.

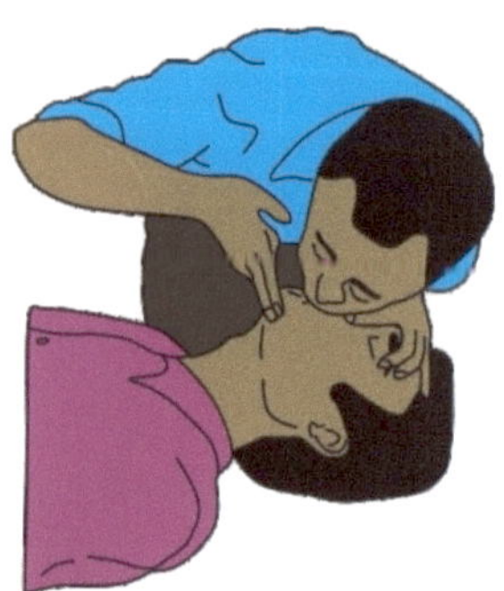

B.   <u>B</u>reathing
The best way to give rescue breathing is by using the mouth-to-mouth technique.

Using the thumb and forefinger of your hand that's on the victim's forehead, pinch the person's nose shut. Be sure to keep the heel of your hand in place so the person's head remains tilted backwards. Keep your other hand under the person's chin, lifting up.

Make an air-tight seal with your mouth on the victim's mouth, then immediately give two full breaths.

C.   Circulation
After giving two full breaths, find the person's carotid artery pulse to see if the heart is still beating.

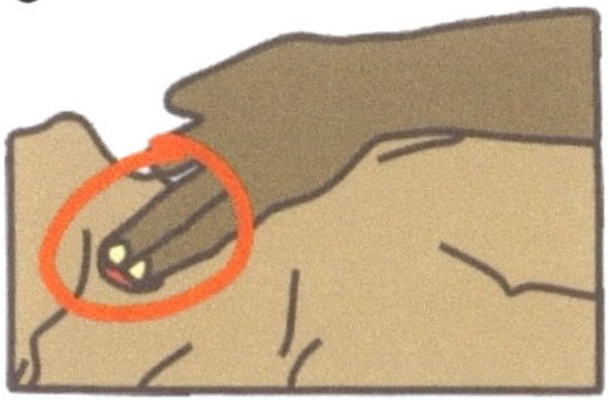

To find the carotid artery pulse, take your hand that's lifting the chin and find the person's Adam's apple (voice box). Slide the tips of your fingers over to the grove beside the Adam's apple and feel for the pulse (heartbeat). If you can't find a pulse, besides providing rescue breathing, you will have to also provide artificial circulation.

Chest Compressions
These provide artificial circulation. When you apply rhythmic pressure on the lower half of the victim's breastbone, you force the heart to pump blood.

To do external chest compression properly:
- Kneel beside the victim's chest.
- With the middle and index fingers of your hand nearest the person's legs, find the notch where the bottom rims of the two halves of the rib cages meet in the middle of the chest. That is the sternum.
- Put the heel of your one hand on the sternum (breastbone) next to

the fingers that found the notch.
- Place your other hand on top of the hand that is in position.
- Be sure to keep your fingers up off the chest wall. It may be easier to do this if you interlock your fingers.
- Bring your shoulders directly over the victim's sternum and press down, keeping your arms straight.
- If the victim is an adult, depress the sternum about 1 and a half or 2 inches; then completely relax the pressure on the sternum. Do not remove your hands from the victim's sternum, but do let the chest rise back to its normal position between compressions. Note that relaxation and compression should take equal amounts of time.

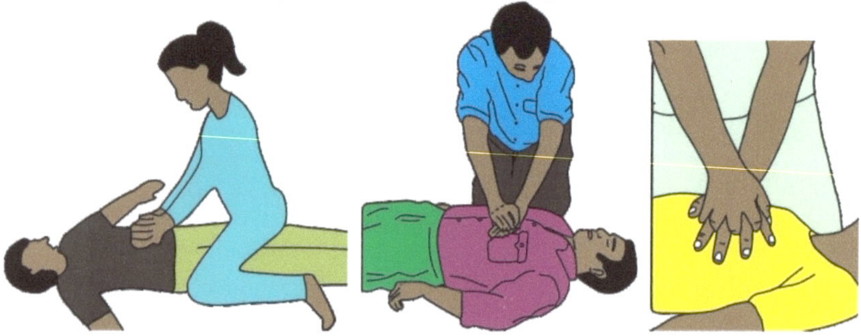

If you must give both rescue breathing and external chest compressions, the proper rate is 15 chest compressions to 2 breaths. You must compress at a rate of 80 to 100 times per minute.

Neck Injury

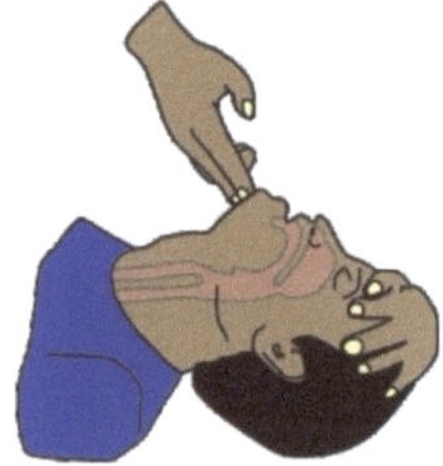

If you suspect that the victim may have a neck injury (such as might occur in a diving or automobile accident for example), you must open the airway differently.

- Open the airway using a chin-lift without tilting the head.
- If the airway stays blocked, tilt the head slowly and gently until the airway is open.

For Infants (Birth to 1 year) and Children (1 to 8 years)
Cardiopulmonary resuscitation for infants and children is similar to that for adults, but there are a few important differences. They are given below.

Assessment and Activation

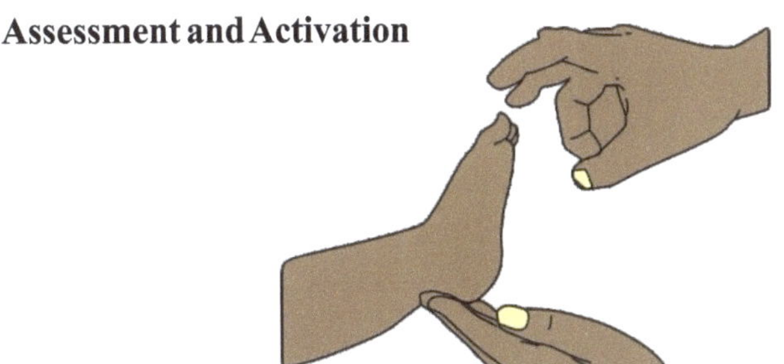

Tap/stroke the child's heel for resonse

If you don't get a response from an infant or child, activate help and begin CPR. If you are alone, do one minute of CPR before leaving to make the necessary call yourself. Return to the victim and continue CPR until help (EMS) arrives or victim is taken to the hospital.

A. **A̲irway**

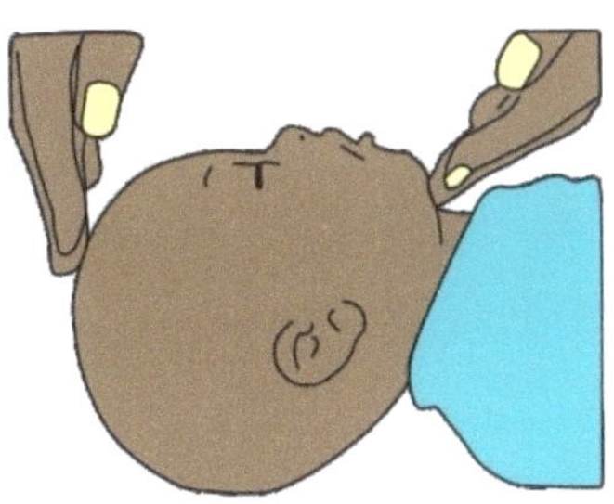

Be careful when handling an infant. Do not tilt the head back too far. An infant's neck bends so easily that if the head is tilted back too far, the breathing passages may be blocked instead of opened.

B.   <u>B</u>reathing

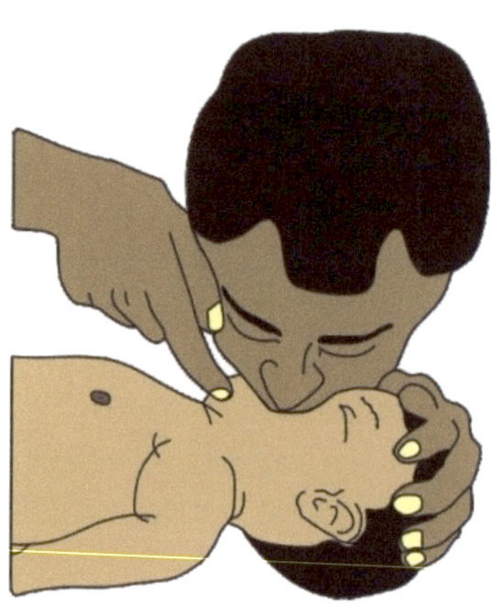

If an infant is not breathing, do not try to pinch the nose shut. Cover both the mouth and nose firmly with your mouth and breathe slowly (1.0 to 1.5 seconds per breath). Use enough volume and pressure to make the chest rise. With a small child, pinch the nose, cover the mouth and breathe the same as for an Infant.

C.   <u>C</u>irculation

In an infant, check for a pulse (heartbeat) by feeling on the inside of the upper arm midway between the elbow and the shoulder. Check for the pulse in a small child the same way you would in an adult.

Chest Compressions

- In infants and small children, use only one hand for compression. You can slip your other hand under the back of an infant to give firm support.
- For **infants**, use only the tips of the middle and ring fingers to compress the chest at the sternum (breastbone). A summary of information is given in the table below. Depress the sternum

between $^{1}/_{2}$ to 1 inch at a rate of at least 100 times a minute.
- For **small children**, use only the heel of one hand (see table for position). Depress the sternum between 1 and & 1½ inches, depending on the child's size. The rate should be 100 times a minute.
- In the case of both infants and small children, give breath during a pause after every fifth chest compression.

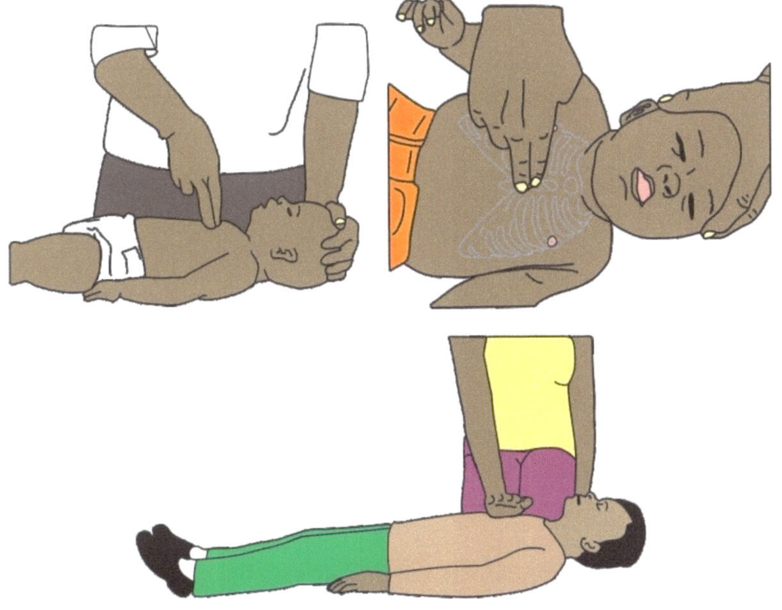

	Part of Hand	Hand Position	Depress Sternum	Rate of Compression
Infants	Tips of middle and ring fingers	1 finger's width below line between nipples	½ to 1 inch	At least 100 times per minute
Children	Heel of hand	Sternum (the same as adults)	1 to 1½ inches	100 times per minute

* Be sure not to depress the tip of the sternum

Remember:

A.   <u>A</u>irway -
Is the victim unresponsive? If so, call for help, position the child and open the airway.

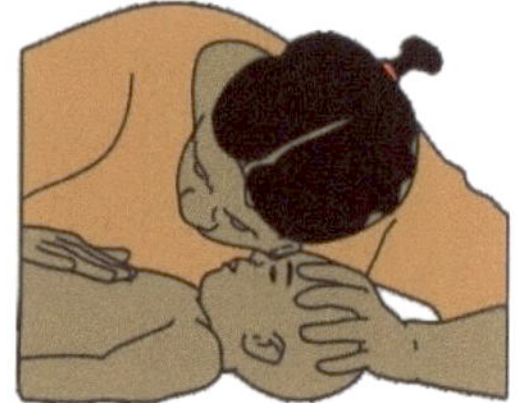

B.   <u>B</u>reathing -
Check for breathing. If there is no breathing, give 2 full breaths. Look out for chest rise, listen for sound of breathing, feel for breath on your cheek.

C.   <u>C</u>irculation -
If the victim is still not breathing, attempt to check the pulse for a few seconds. If there is no pulse and the child is still unresponsive, begin 1 minute of CPR. Then leave to get someone else to get help or you make the necessary call yourself. Continue with the CPR until help arrives.

If the child responds, roll him/her over to the recovery position.

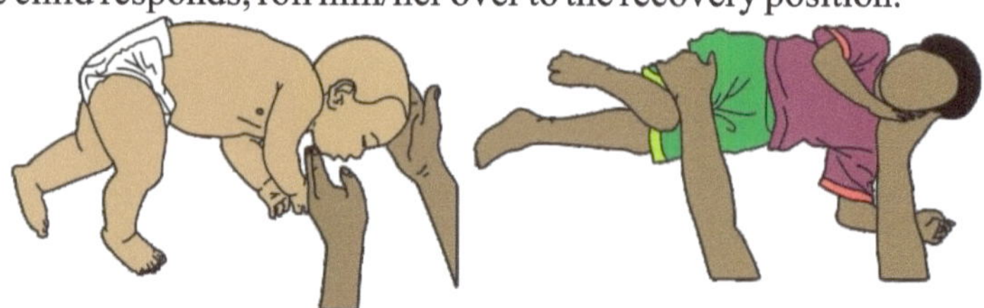

Alternate compressions and rescue breathing at the proper ratio:
- CPR for children over 8 years old is the same as for adults.
- CPR for children over 8 years old is the same for adults.
- For adults and large children, the ratio is 15 compressions to 2 full breaths at the rate of 80 to 100 compressions a minute.
- For small children, the proper ratio is 5 compressions to 1 full breath at a rate of 100 compressions per minute.
- For infants the proper ratio is 5 compressions to 1 full breath at a rate of 100 compressions per minute.

Continue CPR without stopping until advanced life support is available.

Note Please: Periodic practice in CPR is essential to keep your skills at the level they need to be. Someone's life may depend on how well you remember and - apply - the steps in CPR. Have your CPR skills and knowledge tested at least once a year. It could enable you to save a life: sometimes, it may just be the life of someone you love.

HEIMLICH MANEUVER

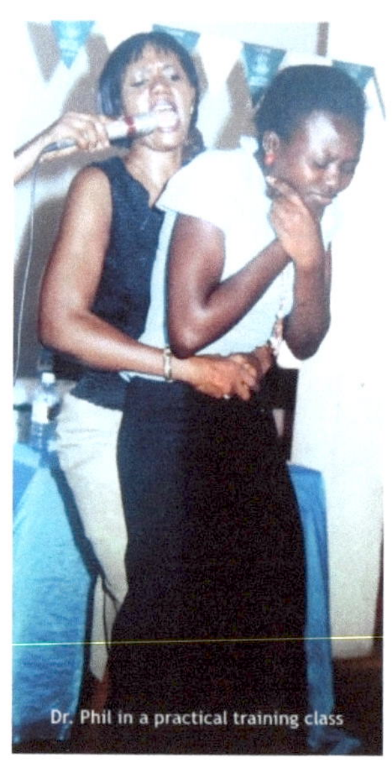
Dr. Phil in a practical training class

Heimlich maneuver is first aid administered when there is an obstruction of the airways in an individual resulting in choking.

Choking occurs when a foreign body finds its way into the throat and blocks the victim's windpipe. With choking, the victim may soon lose consciousness and even die unless there is a prompt rescue operation.

Choking is very serious. Preventing it and knowing the practical skill steps to take in cases of emergency for infants, children and adults is extremely important. Everyone should know the signals of choking and the actions for survival. They should also have a plan for emergency action.

Recognizing a Victim of Choking
A foreign object that is stuck at the back of the throat may block the airway or cause a muscular spasm. If blockage of the airway is partial, the victim

should be able to clear it by him or herself. If the blockage is complete, she/he will be unable to speak, breathe or cough. The victim with the lack of breathing, may also soon lose consciousness.

The rescuer should be prepared to begin rescue breathing and chest compressions (as in Cardiopulmonary Resuscitation *CPR*) in the event of the victim's sudden death. The throat muscles may also relax, leaving the airways sufficiently open for rescue breathing.

Adults, children and infants can choke on food, meat or fishbone. Young children are most prone to choking. A child may choke on food, or may put small objects like buttons or sweets into the mouth thereby causing a blockage of the airway. A drunken person may also choke on his or her own vomit, or during hiccups if there is a foreign object in the mouth.

Other conditions that may cause a blocked airway and possible unconsciousness include stroke, epilepsy, head injury, alcoholic intoxication, drug overdose, swelling from infection and coma.

In most cases the victim gets rapidly distressed and you will need to act quickly to clear any obstruction, if not the victim may lose consciousness.

Choking is very serious. Preventing it and knowing the first aid steps for infants, children and adult victims is extremely important.

Recognition:
With Partial Obstruction –
- There will be coughing and distress
- There will difficulty in speaking

With Complete Obstruction –
- There will be inability to speak, breathe or cough
- There will be obvious distress
- There will be an eventual loss of consciousness

Rescuer's Aims:
- To remove the obstruction immediately where possible

- To arrange to take the victim to the hospital immediately if necessary.

WARNING -
If at any stage the victim becomes unconscious, open the airway and give CPR as explained earlier and ensure you get him/her to the nearest hospital as soon as possible.

Steps to Take:
- If the victim is breathing, encourage him or her to continue coughing. Remove any obvious obstruction from the mouth.
- If the victim becomes weak, or stops breathing or coughing, carry out back slaps.
- Stand slightly by the side behind victim. Support victim's chest with one and help him/her to lean well forward.
- Using the heel of your hand, give victim 5 sharp back slaps between the shoulder blades. Stop if the obstruction clears and sweep the victim's mouth with a clean finger.

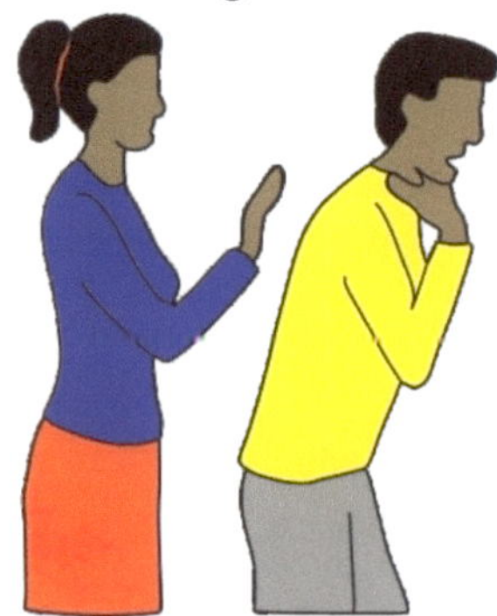

If back slaps fail to clear the obstruction, then try abdominal thrusts **(Heimlich Maneuver)**
- Stand behind victim and straddle his/her legs
- Put your hands around the upper part of victim's abdomen

- Ensure victim is bending well forwards
- Clench your fist and place your thumb inwards between the navel and the bottom of the breastbone
- With your other hand still grasping your fist, pull sharply inwards and upwards up to five times.
- Alternate 5 back slaps and 5 abdominal thrusts until the object of choking is dislodged.

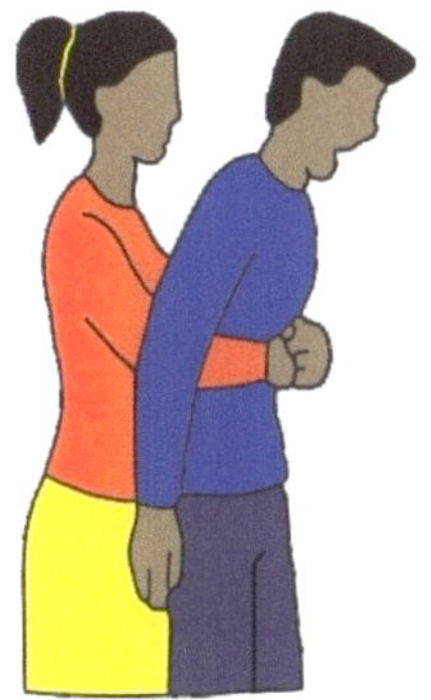

If victim is a child, pregnant or obese, apply **chest thrusts** as against abdominal thrusts.

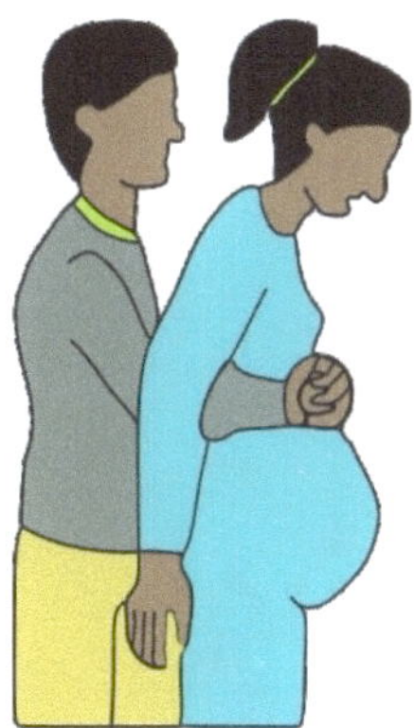

Steps to take for infants (under 1 year old)
- Confirm obstruction of the airways: if baby cannot make sounds, or breathe, or cry or cough while in obvious distress;

- Support baby's neck with one arm and position him/her face down with head lower than body;
- Apply 5 back thrusts between shoulder blades with one hand.
- Turn baby over, still supporting neck with your arm and apply 5 chest thrusts using 2-3 fingertips; compress about 1" deep;
- Repeat several times until the cause of the choking loosens up;
- If the choking object does not come loose or the baby becomes unconscious, commence CPR until medical help is accessed.

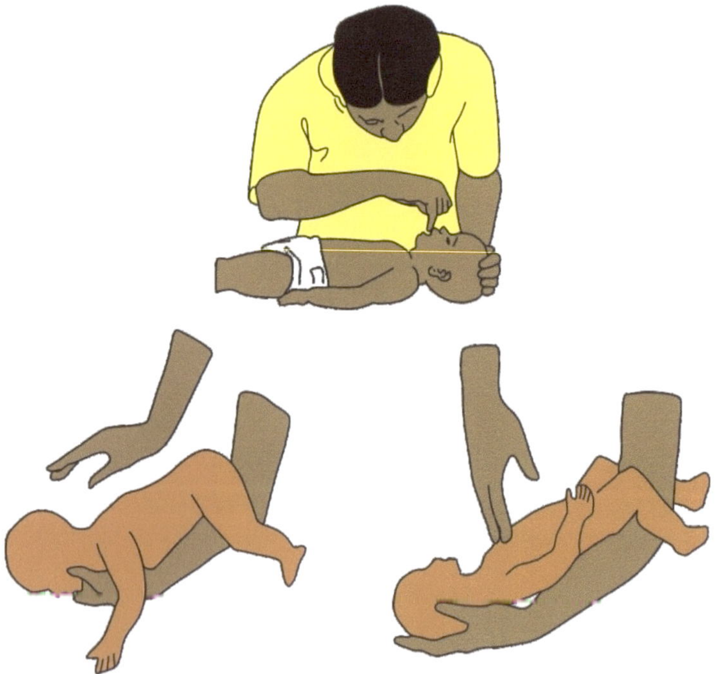

In all cases, look in mouth from time to time to check for and remove choking object if visible and be prepared to take victim to the hospital.

DANGERS OF STRESS AND DEPRESSION

Stress and depression have many health dangers including ultimate death from cardiovascular ailments.

Stress:
Attitude is everything while talking about stress. When you are upset, unhappy, over excited, angry, self-blaming, very tired, jealous, covetous, depressed or suffering from a traumatic experience, then you are most likely DISTRESSED.

When this happens, there is a contraction in your arteries even without you knowing it. When a man or woman feels so hurt that he/she allows the sun to set and rise on a worry, a message is sent to the brain - the body's processor which in turn processes and analyzes it before sending hormones down to the heart.

The sympathetic nervous system will then come in to help you fight or fly away. It will position itself to aid you in whichever decision you make for example: When a man is running for his dear life from danger, he exhibits certain traits that are surprising even to himself. It is the sympathetic nervous system that actually did the trick.

Therefore, when the very smart brain detects a very angry intention, the hormones that are sent to the heart also convey the anger message. There is a sudden change in the heartbeat rate. The beat becomes quite irregular and more blood is pumped ready for the fight or flight subconscious action. More glucose and energy are also produced by the body all set for the fight.

Due to these, the level of a dead hormone known as cortisone is increased. Cortisone is over the adrenaline gland and the kidney inside a human body. When cortisone is triggered, it shows up in the blood and causes the platelet (i.e. the hormone responsible for clotting in the event of an injury to the body) to increase inside the body ready to clot blood should there be a cut, so as to stop the victim from rapidly bleeding to death. If at the end of the day there was no cut on your body but you are still angry, the platelet

will not go back to source. It will rather cling on to the walls of your artery. As time goes on, it forms a blood clot within your arteries. The longer the anger subsists, the more cortisone (the dead or stress hormone) is triggered.

Excess stress and cortisone level in the arteries can lead to a situation where there is an unnecessary obstruction to normal blood flow in the body (arterial contraction). This is because the body wants to conserve what it has for supply in the case of an injury.

If you calm down right after the initial wave of anger, forgetting or letting go of your worries, the parasympathetic nervous system immediately retires and the cortisone level comes down again. This is why it is important for us not allow our anger, anxiety, sleeplessness or frustrations last longer than is necessary. Otherwise, the blood is forced to pass through the arterial contraction resulting in the sick condition known as hypertension (High Blood Pressure).

Hemoglobin carries oxygen from the heart back to the brain, so if there is a high pressure in the flow of blood, the oxygen supply to the brain is reduced (the brain cannot survive without oxygen for more than six minutes). If and when the brain is starved of adequate oxygen, the patient soon develops a nagging headache. This is why there's always the complaint of splitting headaches in most hypertension cases.

When the hypertension patient fails to effectively control the high blood pressure, other vital organs in the body like the kidney, the heart, the pancreatic organ through which insulin is released, the eyes and brain all begin to suffer. Soon they become diseased and the cells start dying.

It is noteworthy that patients of High B.P. have the tendency to easily suffer stroke or develop other health problems like brain hemorrhage, hypertrophy, renal (kidney) damage, myocardial infarction, diabetes, eye problems like cataract, retinopathy, etc. Slowly the patient too begins to die.

Depression:
Depression is characterized by both physical and psychological symptoms. It is not just simply a low mood or sign of personal weakness. It is a common condition that can be safely and effectively treated. People often fail to recognize the symptoms of depression in themselves or people they care about. The first step towards defeating depression is to define it.

Symptoms of Depression
- Overwhelming sadness
- Loss of interest in sex, exercise and pleasurable activities
- Insomnia or oversleeping
- Loss/increase in appetite
- Feelings of hopelessness
- Feelings of worthlessness
- Difficulty concentrating
- Fatigue
- Delusions
- Thoughts of suicide

If five or more of these symptoms are present every day for at least two weeks and interfere with routine daily activities, one should seek professional evaluation or treatment for depression.

Many cases of depression emerge from decreased activity of a particular neurotransmitter or over activity of the hormonal system. Hormones released by the pituitary gland control release of stress hormones in other organs. The chronic activation of the adrenaline glands alters the body's response to stress.

Cardiac patients with depression have an increased risk of blood clotting due to an increase in platelet activity. Increased stress hormones may lead to heart disease and gastrointestinal problems. Untreated depression has a negative impact on the person's physical health, which further deteriorates mental well-being.

There is also the manic-depressive illness which is also called bipolar

disorder. It is characterized by cycling mood changes. A cycle of depression can be followed by a manic phase as the individual becomes overactive with delusions of grandeur, and engages in potentially self-destructive activities. Mania, if untreated, may worsen to a psychotic state.

Depression decreases one's feeling of self-worth and increases the risk of suicide.

Gender differences:
- Women experience depression twice as often as men. This may be due to hormonal factors such as menstrual changes, pregnancy, miscarriage or menopause. Sensitivity to certain changes in the environment may also play a part.
- Men's depression is often masked by alcoholism, drugs or working excessively long hours.
- Individuals who have a family history of depression and a traumatic childhood also seem to be unusually prone to depression.

Treatment for Depression:
Although depression is a common illness, only a fraction of those affected seek or receive treatment. Depression can be safely treated with psychotherapy, medications, or a combination of both.

- Cognitive therapies target thinking patterns.
- Interpersonal therapy targets negative feelings and relationship-based issues.

- Drug treatments are designed to correct the imbalance of chemical messages between the nerve cells and the brain.

Please Note Importantly:
Depression is an illness that can recur, and may require long term treatment. Note also that drug treatments for depression are not addictive.

HEADACHE

Headache is not a disease; it is only a warning sign from your body that all might not be well; that there could be some other underlining problems that may need looking into.

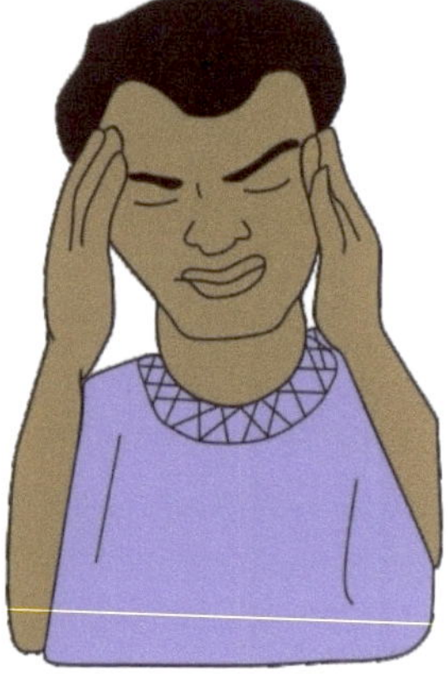

A headache may accompany any illness, particularly a feverish ailment like flu. Of course, it can also come for no reason but can often be traced to tiredness, tension, or stress.

Apart from Stress, several other situations can also cause a headache like starvation arising from dry fasting, an irregular feeding pattern, an infection within the body, or undue heat or cold. It can also be caused by mild "poisoning" from a stuffy or fume-filled atmosphere, excess alcohol, or any other drug.

It may also be the most prominent symptoms of meningitis or stroke. Some people even suffer from more sickening headaches known as migraine.

As we grow older, duties or habits like dry fasting begin to tell on us. Our bodies gradually begin to reject the practice since it means a starvation of the cells. It becomes necessary therefore that we should at least drink a glass of water during our fasting. The reason for drinking water is to help thin the blood so that it can flow freely through its normal channels.

A woman once ran up to me to thank me for my T.V program on the Nigerian Television Authority (N.T.A). She narrated how our edition on Prevention and Remedies for Nagging Headaches had saved her life. According to her she had frequently suffered from headaches for some years now, but that when she tried the tips I provided on the program, the headaches left and has for long not bothered her again. I praised God with her on that day and enjoin you now to take advantage of these life-saving tips.

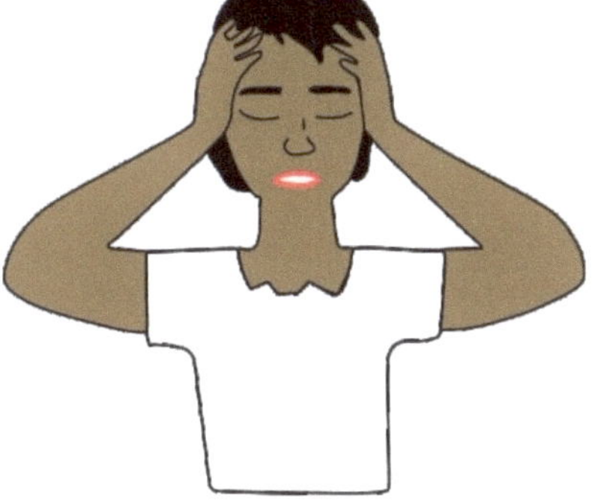

When you feel a headache, it is important that you ask yourself the following questions: Have I taken any water today? Have I eaten something today? Have I over worked myself today and perhaps need a rest? Whatever be the case, just go ahead and drink a glass of water first of all to at least feed the cells; then stop whatever you are doing and rest awhile.

NOTE: When a healthy person is resting, the heart relaxes; but if we are at work, the heart works even harder. Normally when we rest, the heart just has to pump only about 5 liters of blood per minute. During strenuous work or exercises, the same adult's heart pump approximately 25 liters of blood each minute.

When you have rested, the next step to take if the headache still subsists is not to take a pain reliever. Pain killers just shield off a nerve around the medulla oblongata. This stops you momentarily from feeling the headache while the underlining source of the headache remains, ready to resurface another time.

Instead, you will be better off to take some vitamins like Vitamin 'B' Complex or a blood tonic to increase the hemoglobin that is sent to the head. B complex is known to calm the nerves. If and when all these attempts fail, then it may be time to take your pain killer and then see a doctor for further diagnosis.

HIGH BLOOD PRESSURE (HYPERTENSION)

Hypertension kills slowly and silently. Many have died from its terrible consequences. Be warned!

In adults above 30 years, recurrent headaches may be time to assess your blood pressure to ascertain your status. The ideal blood pressure in young adults is 120/70. As you get older from 25 years, the pressure may increase to like 125/75 or 135/80 etc. This is as a direct consequence of the rising level of stress and various toxins introduced into our systems through various kinds of food be it alcohol, cholesterol, saturated animal fat and other junk meals.

The stress and toxins gradually cause a buildup of plaques in the arteries resulting in a narrowing of the channel for the free flow of blood. As this worsens with age, the flow of blood becomes more pressured. It is therefore pertinent that younger people take advantage of the information and cultivate healthier feeding habit as an insurance against an unhealthy older age.

When a young adult's blood pressure exceeds 140/90 the border line, hypertension can be said to have set in. In adults above 45 years with high level deposit of plaques in the arteries, the blood pressure level may reach 145/95 but if it reaches 150/100 you need professional attention immediately. If the patient fails to heed this warning, then there is a high tendency for him/her to suffer a stroke or just slump and die suddenly as a result of one cardiovascular affliction or the other.

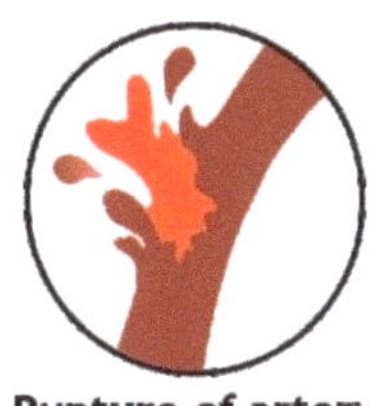

Rupture of artery

CAUSES, EFFECTS & REMEDIES FOR CARDIOVASCULAR DISEASES

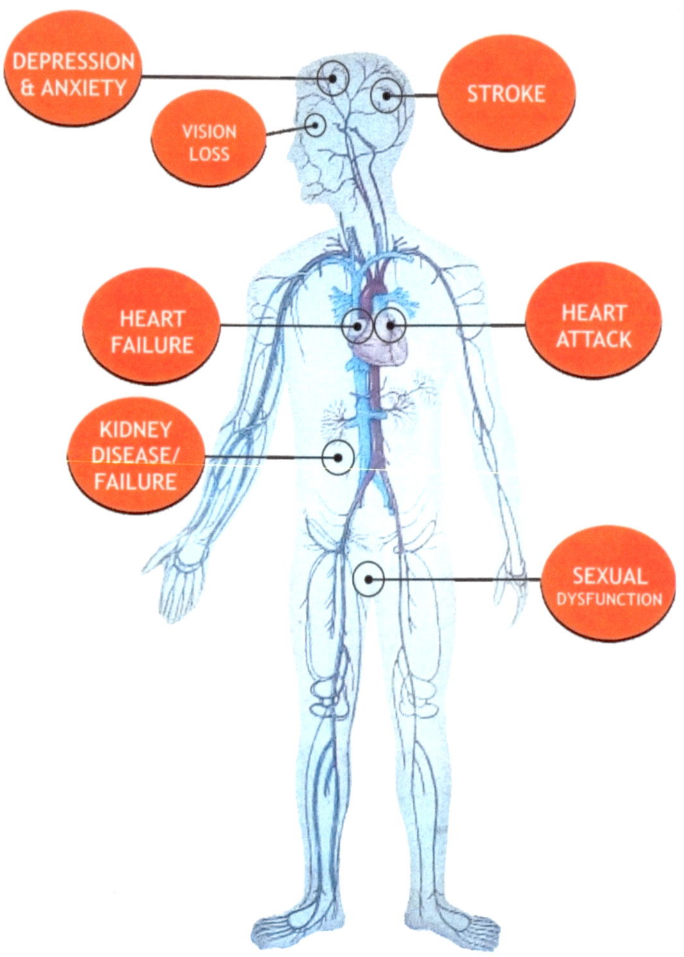

Our body comprises of wires and tube like network / circuit that is otherwise known as the nerves and arteries. Some of this "wires" carry electrical impulses through the body while the tubes are channels for the free flow of both oxygenated and de-oxygenated blood.

When one is so anxious or angry that you do not let go when you should, there is a contraction of the arteries obstructing the free flow of blood, and then there is the danger of the platelet released during this period of distress to form a blood clot within the walls of the arteries.

If the "tube" that carries blood from the heart to the rest of the body also known as the coronary artery is completely obstructed by the formation of a clot, then a portion of the heart muscle dies (see illustration below).

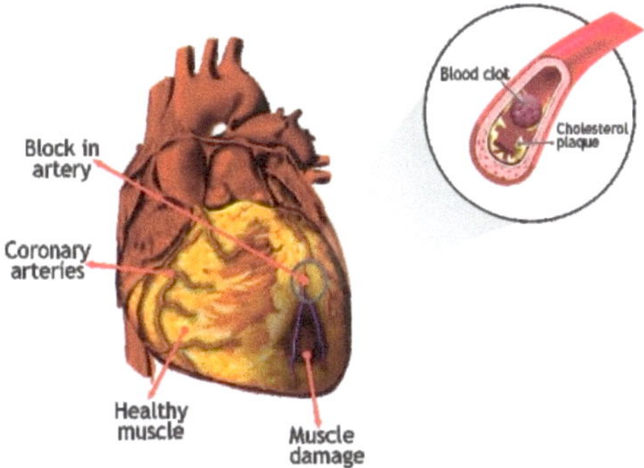

The diagrams below describe what a blood clot or plaque looks like in the artery. If you look closely, you will notice that the clot or cholesterol plaque would ordinarily obstruct the free flow of blood to vital organs.

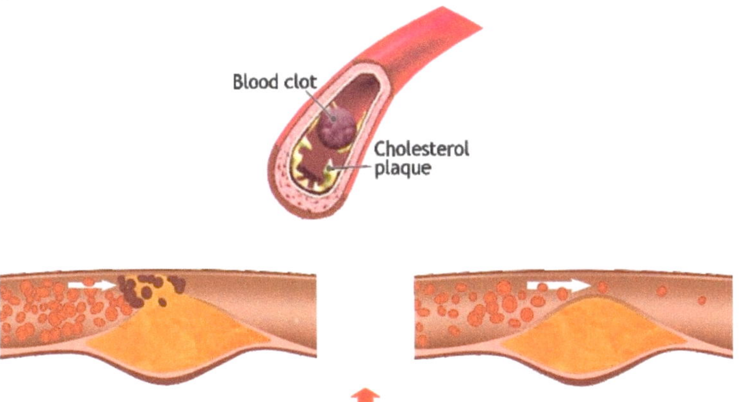

Blood clot and cholesterol plaque build-up in the artery

When a portion of the heart muscle dies as a result of the obstruction or plaque, there is a discoloration of the area and a small pain may be felt in the chest around the area belying the heart. As this is happening, the patient notices an irregularity in his heart beat rate and soon, a recurrent chest pain is developed.

Of course, the patient may also then develop a condition known as myocardial infarction, a case of an attack to the heart. Soon the pain from the chest area spreads over to the shoulder, neck, back and arms. It is important the patient sees a professional medical practitioner immediately at this point to be assessed.

When a much larger portion of the heart muscles die, the patient experiences a serious heart attack. Sometimes the first major attack is easily brought under control; but a second could prove very fatal. If the patient is still careless about the condition, then cardiac arrest will occur and the heart will stop pumping. When this happens the patient stops breathing and soon dies.

In most cases, the victim did not even know what he suffered from, while relatives would speculatively conclude that he was struck dead by a spirit or an enemy given the suddenness of the victim's demise.

If the blood clot gets to the carotid artery, there is a partial occlusion of the artery and blood will no longer flow freely into the affected part of the head. The brain cells will start dying and the patient will develop a weakness in that side of the body (left or right). This is the onset of a stroke.

If the left or right carotid artery is completely blocked by the clot, the patient will suffer a partial stroke. If the patient still remains careless about the situation, the clot might also affect the other carotid artery. This time, the patient will suffer a complete stroke and may become quadriplegic.

To Prevent Blood Clots in the Arteries:
- Do not worry
- Be happy and laugh always
- Exercise regularly

To Prevent Plaque Build-up in the Arteries:
- Avoid oils like the palm oil we use in cooking. Palm oil contains a lot of fat and I urge you not to eat too much of it. Instead eat more of palm nut sauces.
- Stay away from all groundnut/vegetable oils that congeal under low temperature. You are better off with zero or low cholesterol oils.
- Avoid fried foods as much as possible. Cooked, baked or broiled foods are always better.
- Avoid eating the egg yolk; it contains a high level of the cholesterol dangerous to your body. You can try eating the egg white alone.
- Check your cholesterol level regularly.
- Avoid the fat from the chicken skin, remove all the fat from your meal before eating (i.e. if you must eat meat). Red meat becomes an enemy to our body, as we grow older. The entrails of animals are exceptionally good as seasoning or stock for our sauce; but it is poison to us, as it is fatty and oily.
- Reduce your intake of alcohol. Alcohol has fat and also causes a contraction in the arteries.
- Stay away from tobacco smoking and smoke.
- Generally, be careful of what you eat; it's healthier to eat more of fruits and vegetable.

Remedies:
If you are above 45 years old and have experienced cases of high blood pressure, stroke, blood clotting or plaque buildup, then this is for you.

Aspirin is the wonder drug to beat if taken after a meal (note: not for ulcer patients). It thins the blood and allows it to flow more freely through the arteries to the brain and to the vital organs. Be sure to take one tablet of aspirin at least three times or more a week only at night after meals and once daily for all stroke survivors.

It is life saving for all high blood pressure patients to be placed on aspirin. However, as research   suggests stroke survivors should not stop taking the daily dose of aspirin as this might triple the risk of another stroke within a month.

WARNING! Be Careful -
- Taking Ibuprofen around the same time you are taking aspirin, counteracts the benefits of taking aspirin to prevent heart disease. Usually, doing this increases the risk of fatal illness in the patient.
- Ulcer patients MUST NOT take aspirin until the ulcer is effectively treated.
- Taking Aspirin and Vitamin E at the same time can cause bleeding as Vitamin E also thins the blood.
- Aspirin should only be taken after meals at night, when the body is expected to rest.

Whatsoever situation you find yourself, there's only one thing to do:

Laugh and be happy!

That is the world's best remedy to the worst of all situations.

www.ingramcontent.com/pod-product-compliance
Lightning Source LLC
Chambersburg PA
CBHW040233240726
48664CB00001B/112